Food for Pregnancy Volume 3

The Mom's Guide to Understanding the Best Supplements and Nutrients for a Healthy Growing Baby

MIA ANGLES

Table of Contents

acknowledge that the author is not engaging in the rendering of legal, financial, medical or professional advice. The content of this book has been derived from various sources. Please consult a licensed professional before attempting any techniques outlined in this book.

By reading this document, the reader agrees that under no circumstances is the author responsible for any losses, direct or indirect, which are incurred as a result of the use of information contained within this document, including, but not limited to, —errors, omissions, or inaccuracies.

Introduction

I want to thank you for choosing the book, '*Food for Pregnancy Volume 3 - The Moms Guide to Understanding the Best Supplements and Nutrients for a Healthy Growing Baby*'

The first two volumes of the book provided information on the different types of food that you are allowed to eat. Those volumes helped you understand why it was important for you to watch your diet during your pregnancy. This book will discuss something a little more important.

You are bound to be under immense stress during pregnancy, and this will lead to some issues during labor or after pregnancy. It is extremely important that you understand how to deal with this stress. This book sheds some light on why women may be under undue stress during pregnancy, and also provides some tips that you can use to overcome that stress. You will also gather information about some toxins that you should be wary of, and what you should do to avoid any exposure to those toxins.

You have taken care of yourself and have given birth to a healthy new baby. Now, what do you do? How do you care for your body? This book will shed some light on the different changes you can expect in your body, and also talks about how you can handle those changes. I hope the information in this book will help you go through pregnancy with ease.

Chapter One: Toxins to Avoid During Pregnancy

When you are pregnant, you are advised to avoid alcohol and to stop smoking. Research shows that consumption of alcohol during pregnancy can lead to fetal alcohol syndrome, and smoking increases the risk of stillbirth, sudden infant death syndrome and miscarriage. It does seem a bit strange when people ask you to give up on using nail polish, using air freshener or drinking water from plastic bottles doesn't it? Research conducted by the Environmental Working Group (EWG) shows that the chemicals in these products are not safe for you or your baby, and they can be as toxic as alcohol or smoke. The chemicals present in these products will get into your blood stream and will pass to the fetus through the placenta. If these toxins are passed through to the fetus during the developmental stages, it can cause irreversible or permanent organ and brain damage. This damage will not just be present at birth but will continue into adulthood.

The research conducted by EWG concluded that a baby could be born with close to 232 industrial pollutants and compounds. Some of these pollutants and compounds are found in water and soil, and it is impossible to avoid them. There are others that can be found in house paint and shampoos, and it is easy to avoid these. This chapter lists ten pollutants that you should protect yourself and your baby from.

Lead

Lead is a powerful neurotoxic metal known to cause nervous system disorders, permanent brain damage, hyperactivity and learning and behavior difficulties. If you are exposed to this metal during your pregnancy, you may endanger your child. Lead is known to slow down the growth of a child, both in the uterus and after their birth.

How do you think exposure occurs? You may drink water from the tap, and this water may be contaminated with lead. Lead contaminates water if the pipes are maintained poorly or the metal is very old. This is what happened in a city in Michigan. You may also inhale some dust tainted with lead from chipping or old paint. You could be working in a garden where the soil is contaminated by lead because of a building that was last painted in the year 1978. Lead was banned from paints only after 1978. There are some lipsticks that have some lead in them because the pigments used to give the lipstick some color contain lead.

How to Avoid Lead

You should ensure that the tap that you use for water is free of lead. You should check the Consumer Confidence Report issued by the water utility in your area. If the tap water not free of lead, you should contact the officials in your area and demand that they repair the water system in the area. Alternatively, you can purchase a filter that will filter any contaminants, including lead, from the water.

If your house was built before the year 1978, you should use a test kit and verify if the paint is free of lead or not. The results of your test will tell you if you need to call a lead-abatement specialist. If you want to renovate an older home, you should vacate the residence and move to a lead-free area. If you do want to use cosmetics, you should stick to using organic products where the pigments used are natural fruit pigments.

Mercury

Mercury is another neurotoxic that will impede the development of the brain and nervous system. The mercury that we are exposed to is through air pollution. When a power plant burns coal, it releases mercury into the air, which then falls into fresh water lakes, rivers, streams and oceans. It will then accumulate in fish like shark, tilefish, king mackerel, swordfish and tuna. Mercury is also present in older thermometers and fluorescent light bulbs, but the highest exposure comes through seafood that has mercury in it.

How to Avoid Mercury

As mentioned in the previous books, you should consume seafood that is low in mercury, but rich in omega-3 fatty acids, like tilapia, anchovies, shrimp, cod, pollock, trout and sardines. You should also switch to using a digital thermometer or use a CFL bulb or LED bulb, as these are energy efficient.

PCBs

PCBs or polychlorinated bisphenols were labeled as possible human carcinogens by the U. S. Environmental Protection Agency (EPA). PCBs also damage the human immune, neurological and reproductive systems. These compounds have been banned since the year 1976, but they can still be found in animals and people who live near areas where PCBs used to be produced.

People often ingest PCBs through food. As mentioned earlier, soil may get contaminated because of PCBs. Cattle that graze on this soil will be contaminated with PCBs. Studies conducted by researchers in the state of Washington found that there were high levels of PCBs in the packaging of some foods like macaroni and cheese, taco shells, cheese and cracker snack packs and more. PCBs are also used in inks and coloring, and have been found in magazines, house paints and newspapers.

How to Avoid PCBs

Studies show that PCBs are found in large quantities in fat, and it is for this reason that you should avoid consuming fatty fish and red meat. You should always trim the fat from any of the foods that you eat. It is a good idea to consume grains, organic fruit and vegetables instead of consuming processed food. You should also switch to non-toxic primers and paints.

Formaldehyde

Formaldehyde is a pollutant that is found in most products, especially household products like cabinets, furniture made from pressed wood, chairs, couches and other furniture, fabric softeners and carpeting. This pollutant is also used in shampoos, nail polishes and cosmetics as a preservative. People are often exposed to formaldehyde when the chemical evaporates from the product it is in and mixes with the air. Studies show that formaldehyde has negative effects on the immune system. Studies conducted on lab animals showed that formaldehyde will lead to low birth weight.

How to Avoid Formaldehyde

It is important that you read the labels carefully and only purchase those products that are free of formaldehyde. If you do want to use nail polish, you should choose those products that are free of formaldehyde and other chemicals. Make sure that you always paint your nails in a well-ventilated room. If you are installing cabinets or carpets in your house, make sure that you leave your windows open.

Always purchase cabinets that are made fully of wood instead of purchasing products that are made using particleboards or pressed wood. Do not use air fresheners with aerosol, atomized perfume and plug-in fragrance dispensers.

Phthalates

Plastic is often softened using a chemical compound called a phthalate. These chemicals make it easy for companies to make smooth body lotion, prevent the hair spray from getting stiff and also make nail polish easy to apply. If you use capsules, there is a possibility that you may consume phthalates. These chemicals are also used to deliver fragrances. They are used in household cleaning products, perfumes, commercial air fresheners, personal care products and detergents to release their smells.

Studies were conducted on male lab animals to understand the effects of phthalates on males. These studies concluded that phthalates can lead to decreased sperm count, infertility, malformations of the urethra and penis and undescended testes. Studies conducted by the National Institutes of Health concluded that phthalates reduced the chances of pregnancy in women, and these studies also showed that children who were born to women who were exposed to phthalates during their pregnancy were at a higher risk of developing ADHD. These babies may also be born with a low birth weight, may be born prematurely or may be susceptible to becoming overweight later in life.

How to Avoid Phthalates

Make sure you always read labels. You should always substitute the air fresheners that are made with synthetic fragrances, including plug-in air fresheners, hanging car air fresheners, air sprays with fragrances with phthalate-free products. You should always use fewer personal care products since your skin absorbs the chemicals from the different products you use. You should avoid microwaving any food in a plastic container since the phthalates from the plastic will move into the food. You should also avoid using vinyl raincoats and shower curtains since vinyl also contains phthalates.

Flame Retardants

Polybrominated diphenyl ethers or PBDEs are industrial chemicals used to retard flames especially in furniture, plastic and mattresses. These chemicals can be exposed to the air, soil and water when they are used and manufactured. They are not water soluble, and they tend to settle at the bottom of lakes or rivers, and as a result can accumulate in fish. These chemicals also mix with the house dust. PBDEs will interfere with the metabolism, development of the brain and nervous system and growth. It is for this reason that children who are affected by PBDEs have lower cognitive abilities. PBDEs also contribute to some disease in adults.

How to Avoid PBDEs

PBDEs are used to manufacture foam and upholstery. If you have any old furniture at home, there are chances that the stuffing or the cushion is being exposed. You will need to either cover this or replace the decor to reduce the concentration of PBDEs in the dust. You can also purchase furniture free of PBDEs. Make sure that you choose any electronic made with alternatives to flame-retardants.

Toluene

Toluene is a colorless and a clear liquid with a distinctive smell. This chemical is a good solvent and is used in paint thinners, paints, lacquers, nail polish, rubber, printing, leather tanning processes and adhesives. This chemical is also added to gasoline along with xylene and benzene to improve the ratings of octane. Toluene is often present in the air when there is a lot of traffic. This chemical easily evaporates and is a source of air pollution. If you leave paint or nail polish open for too long, the toluene in the products will evaporate into the air.

Women who are exposed to high levels of toluene during pregnancy are at a higher risk. Toluene can also affect the functions of the liver and kidney, harm the reproductive system and also reduce immunity towards specific diseases. You should ensure that you do not expose yourself to large quantities of toluene.

How to Avoid Toluene

You should always ensure that you purchase those nail polishes that do not have toluene and formaldehyde. You should never refinish or repaint your furniture or refinish your cupboards or banisters when you are pregnant. If you do want to repaint your house, you should use water-based paints. Do not use any paints that you will need to wash off using a paint thinner. If you are filling your car up with gas, make sure that you walk away so you do not inhale the fumes.

PFOS or PFOA

PFOA and PFOS are chemicals that are formulated to produce or manufacture stick and stain resistant. These chemicals are organic compounds that are pre-fluorinated. These compounds are used in fast-food containers, carpeting and furniture, non-stick cooking pans and pots, microwave popcorn bags, pizza boxes and stain resistant clothing. Exposure to pre-fluorinated organic compounds increases the risk of low birth weight. Research is still being conducted to understand the impact that these compounds have on the fetus.

Research conducted in the John Hopkins Bloomberg School of Public Health concluded that pregnant women who had elevated levels of these compounds in their birth gave birth to children who had low weights. These babies also had a smaller head circumference when compared to those babies who were born to women who were not exposed to these chemicals. These conditions led to some medical problems in children later in their lives. Other studies have shown that exposure to these chemicals leads to elevated cholesterol levels, difficulty in conceiving and low sperm quality.

How To Avoid PFOA or PFOS

You should always avoid stain-resistant furniture and ensure that you do not use any stain protection products on your furniture or carpets. You should avoid wearing stain-resistant clothing, and only purchase those clothes that you can launder easily. Make sure that you use napkins when you eat, and never leave any non-stick pots or pans on the gas stove unattended. Never place these pots or pans on high temperatures. If the pans start to deteriorate, you should either get rid of them or replace them with new pots and pans. Try to use seasoned cast iron or stainless-steel cookware.

Asbestos

The compound asbestos is a combination of six fibrous minerals, and research shows that these minerals cause cancer. This material can resist fire, and it is for this reason that this material is used in most parts of the home, including vinyl flooring, attic and pipe insulation, roofing shingles, ceiling tiles, clothing, sheetrock and automotive products like drum brake linings and disc brake pads. The asbestos fibers will be exposed to the air when the products become old, which makes it easy to inhale the chemical. Asbestos is also known to contaminate water because it is found in some rocks and in soil. There are some pre-mixed potting and garden soils that may also have some content of asbestos in them. There is no safe level of exposure to this chemical.

How to Avoid Asbestos

When you are checking the quality of water in your area, make sure that you also check for any asbestos content in the water. Water suppliers are required to adhere to the Safe Drinking Water Act, which states that they will need to remove asbestos from water fully. If it is difficult for them to remove asbestos completely, they should bring the concentration down to 1 MFL. If you see that the report shows that there is a higher concentration, you should meet your city or county representative, and ask them to look into the matter. You should use filters that will help to remove both asbestos and lead from the water.

If you live in a house that was built before the year 1980, you should remember that some of the construction components might be contaminated. You should hire an expert to sample the products in the house and determine the concentration of asbestos. These experts can determine if the items should be removed or if the asbestos can be contained in one place alone. Alternatively, you should hire a certified professional who can clean up the asbestos content in the house. If you love gardening, you should not use vermiculite to improve the quality of the potting soil. You should try to use sawdust, peat, bark or perlite.

Bisphenol A or BPA

Hard polycarbonate plastic used to make bottles, jugs, tableware like cups and plates, food storage containers and baby bottles is made using the petrochemical Bisphenol A or BPA. This compound is also used in thermal cash register receipts and epoxy resin, which is used to line beverage and food cans to prevent any bacterial contamination and corrosion. BPA is a very functional compound, but it is a highly unstable chemical. This compound will leach into the liquids and food from the packaging.

BPA can disrupt the endocrine system in the body, even if it is consumed in small doses. Any exposure to BPA is harmful to the fetus since it can disrupt the development. This chemical increases the risk of developing prostate and breast cancer, changes in gender specific behavior due to changes in brain development and the early onset of puberty. This chemical is also linked to infertility, heart disease, toddler behavior problems, diabetes, erectile dysfunction and miscarriages.

How to Avoid BPA

If you want to decrease your exposure to BPA, you should reduce the number of plastic water bottles you use. You should avoid using the bottles that are labeled as BPA-free. Use aluminum, stainless steel or glass bottles instead. Avoid consuming canned foods and drinks and choose fresh or frozen juices and foods. Instead of consuming carbonated drinks, you should try to drink juices or water out of glass bowls. If you want to eat beans, make sure that you do not buy canned beans. Always soak the beans overnight and cook them before you eat them.

It is difficult to know if a receipt has some BPA in it. So, leave the receipt behind if you are sure that you do not need it. Alternatively, ask the store to email the receipt to you. When you are at the grocery store, you can ask the cashier to drop the receipt in the bag. Remember to never place the receipt in your mouth.

Chapter Two: Stress and Pregnancy

You will notice that your body and your emotions will change during your pregnancy. You will also notice that your life is changing, and so are the lives of every member in your family. You will welcome these changes with happiness, but it is important that you know that these changes will add new stress to your life.

It is common for you to be under a lot of stress during pregnancy. That said, too much stress will make it hard for you to be happy during your pregnancy. You will have headaches, overeat, lose your appetite or even have trouble sleeping.

If you are under high stress for long periods, it will lead to some health problems like high blood pressure and also increase the risk of developing some heart issues. If you are suffering under high stress, you may also give birth earlier than the scheduled date. The chances of low birth weight also increase. If your baby is born too soon or is too small, they are at a higher risk of developing some health problems.

Causes of Stress during Pregnancy

There are different reasons why women are under stress during pregnancy, but there are a few common reasons:

- You may have a backache, nausea, and constipation or feel tired due to pregnancy; it is normal for women to face these discomforts during pregnancy.

- Your mood is bound to change because your hormones keep fluctuating. It becomes very hard for you to handle stress when your mood constantly changes.

- You are probably worried about what can happen during labor or may be worried about how you will care for your child after you give birth.

- If you are working, you are under a lot of pressure to manage your responsibilities and also prepare your colleagues so they can manage your work when you are away from your job.

- It is true that your life may take some unexpected turns, and this is not going to stop because you are pregnant. The changes in your life will affect you and may sometimes cause undue stress.

Types of Stress that Cause Problems during Pregnancy

Every woman is under stress during pregnancy, and if you handle this stress well, you can take on many other challenges. Regular stress like sitting in traffic and work deadlines will not lead to any problems during pregnancy. That said, if you are under undue stress during your pregnancy, the risk of problems like premature birth will increase. Women who are under stress during pregnancy can give birth to healthy babies, but you will need to be careful if you experience the following kinds of stress:

• Negative Life Events

You will be under stress if you lose a job or home or are going through a divorce, some illness or have witnessed a death in the family. These events will lead to immense stress, which can harm you and your baby.

- ### **Catastrophic Events**

Events like terrorist attacks, earthquakes and hurricanes also lead to undue stress.

- ### **Long-lasting Stress**

Long-lasting stress is caused when you are being abused at home or at work, are depressed, are having serious health problems or are facing some financial problems. If you are suffering from depression, you will be upset and sad for long periods making it hard for you to lead a normal life.

- ### **Racism**

Quite a few women face stress caused due to racism. It is for this reason that African-American women are at a higher risk of giving birth to babies with low birth weight or may give birth to babies before the schedules date when compared to women from other ethnic or racial groups.

- ### **Pregnancy Related Stress**

Women are always under stress during their pregnancy, and they add to this stress by constantly worrying about the health of their baby, whether they can handle the pain during labor, how they will be as a parent and about losing their baby. If you find yourself thinking this way, you should speak to your doctor or midwife.

Post-Traumatic Stress Disorder (PTSD) and Pregnancy

PTSD or Post-Traumatic Stress Disorder is when you have trouble after you experience or witness a terrible event like abuse, the loss of a loved one, a natural disaster, a terrorist attack or rape. People who have PTSD may have the following when they are reminded of the event:

- Nightmares

- Flashbacks of the event

- Serious anxiety

- Physical responses like sweating, racing heartbeat and nausea

Almost eight percent of women suffer from PTSD during their pregnancy, and they are likely to give birth to babies with low birth weight or may give birth before the scheduled date when compared to women who do not have PTSD.

Women suffering from PTSD commonly smoke cigarettes, take street drugs or drink alcohol to cope with the anxiety or fear caused due to PTSD. When they behave in this manner, they may have many problems during their pregnancy. If you suffer from PTSD, it is important that you speak to your doctor or midwife and get into contact with a mental health professional who can guide you.

Does stress cause problems during a pregnancy?

Most people do not understand what the effects of stress are on pregnancy. There are some stress-related hormones that can cause numerous complications in pregnancy. Long-lasting stress or serious stress can affect your immune system, and this will increase the chances of developing an infection. Since your immune system is weak, there are chances that you may develop some uterine infections that can lead to premature birth.

Stress will also affect the way you respond to some situations in life. You may start to consume alcohol, or start smoking and may resort to taking street drugs to endure that stress which can lead to some problems in your pregnancy.

How does stress affect your baby later in life?

It is known that high levels of stress can lead to some problems during pregnancy and even after you give birth. Stress affects the development of your child's brain and immune system, and as a result your child may find it hard to pay attention or may be anxious at all times.

Chapter Three: How to Deal with Stress during Pregnancy?

As mentioned earlier, you are bound to be slightly stressed about the numerous changes that are taking place in your body during your pregnancy. If you are only stressed occasionally, you will not have any trouble with your pregnancy. If you are anxious, irritable and stressed throughout the day and for long periods, you should speak to your doctor or midwife to understand why you feel this way. Prolonged or extreme stress can increase the risk of low birth weight. You may not be affected too badly because of the stress that you are under, but it is important that you tackle your issues now so you can enjoy the joys that pregnancy brings.

How to Reduce Stress

Let us look at ten steps that you can take to reduce stress during your pregnancy.

Always Focus On Your Baby

It is important that you take some time out of your busy schedule and focus on yourself. Studies show that it is important for both you and your baby that you relax, so you should never worry about taking some time for yourself. If you have read the books, you know that your baby can hear your voice from the 23rd week, so you should try to sing, read or chat with your baby bump. This is one of the best ways to bond with your child, and you will feel much better about your pregnancy.

Sleep Well

You should always listen to your body. Make sure that you take a nap or go to bed early if you feel too tired. It is also okay to take a break from work if you are tired. Studies show that sleep is important for mental health, and if you are happy, you will have a healthy pregnancy. There are numerous tips that you can use to make sure that you sleep well during your pregnancy.

- Develop a sleep schedule, and make sure that you stick to it. Wake up and go to bed at the same time every day. It is true that you may want to sleep in on some days but remember that when you do that it will be harder for you to sleep at night.

- Get a relaxing massage before bed.
- Create a soothing ritual for yourself before you go to bed. Take a relaxing bath, read a good book or have a warm drink before you get ready for bed.

It is very hard for you to get the rest you need when you become a parent. You still deserve to take some rest. You can always ask your partner, parents, grandparents or friends to look after your child for a few hours so you can have some rest. Take a break for yourself and spend the time doing something you love to do.

Talk about It

If you have any personal problem or are worried about the wellbeing of your baby, you should always talk about it. Speak to your doctor or your midwife about what you are feeling. You should never be afraid of how you truly feel. It is only when you are honest about how you feel that you can get all the support. Your doctor and midwife will have seen so many women go through similar issues and would love to help you overcome your fears instead of letting you suffer in silence. You can also talk to your partner. You may find that your partner is also worried and has some other concerns. It is only when you talk things through that you will feel better about the situation.

If it makes you feel better, you can speak to other pregnant women during an exercise class or a doctor's visit. They may also have the same feelings as you and will want to hear you out.

Eat Well

It is important that you eat well and eat the right food. The food you eat will provide nourishment for your body, your brain and your baby. The first two volumes of the series provided information about the different types of foods you can and cannot eat. You should ensure that you eat meals at regular intervals to ensure that your blood sugar levels do not drop. When your blood sugar levels drop, you will be more irritable and tired.

It is not easy for you to eat well if you do not feel too good about it. If you suffer from morning sickness or nausea, you will avoid food. But you should find a way to consume at least one full meal every day. This will make you feel better. You should also ensure that you drink at least eight glasses of water every day. If you do not consume enough water, you will be dehydrated, and this will affect your mood.

Before you were pregnant, you may have had a glass of wine to help you unwind, but you should avoid alcohol when you are pregnant. You can drink a warm glass of milk instead of wine.

Try Exercise

You may not want to exercise, and this is probably the last thing that will cross your mind, especially when you are pregnant. However, exercise is known to lift a person's spirits at any time. One of the reasons why doctors advise people to exercise is that it helps to release the chemical dopamine in your brain. This chemical is a feel-good chemical. You can do different types of exercises during your pregnancy, and these have been listed in the second volume of the series. You should ensure that you speak to your doctor or midwife before you join any activity. One of the best exercises to do during your pregnancy is swimming. This activity will keep your body toned and will not be too hard on your joints.

You can also join a class for pregnancy yoga. Yoga not only stretches the muscles in your body, but also helps you learn a few meditation techniques that you can use to relax and calm your mind. These techniques will boost your emotional wellbeing. It is a good idea to add a few minutes of exercise to your daily schedule. You can walk around the house as often as you can for ten minutes. If you love being outdoors, you can take a walk in the park.

Prepare For Birth

It is important that you understand what can happen during labor. You should sign up for some classes to understand this better. When you know what you can expect and understand all your options, you will feel confident. It is also a good idea to speak to your doctor or midwife to understand what you can expect from pregnancy, and also ask as many questions as you can. Your doctor or midwife can help you write a plan that will help you define your preferences. There is no harm with making changes to your plan later. It is important that you keep the plan flexible. This will help you remain calm even if the birth does not happen the way you imagined it to.

If you are giving birth in a birth center or a hospital, you can ask your doctor to let you visit the delivery room beforehand. When you are familiar with your surroundings, you will feel better about the whole process and this will help you set your mind to rest. If you are terrified of giving birth and would prefer to have caesarean, you should speak to your doctor or midwife. They can help you handle the fear and anxiety, and also refer you to a therapist who can help you work through your issues. You will feel better about giving birth at the end.

Cope With Commuting

One of the major sources of stress is travel, and this will become worse when you are heavily pregnant. It is unfortunate that your employer only has to worry about work related travel. He is not obligated to think about how you commute to work daily. Having said that, some employers make the effort to help you through your pregnancy and change the shift timings for you, so you do not have to work odd hours or commute during traffic.

It is important for you to keep track of how you sit on public transport. If nobody offers to give you a seat, you can request them to give you one. Pregnant women are given first-class tickets on some trains. You can visit the operator's website to learn more about these tickets.

Sort Out Any Money Issues

Most women worry about how they are going to pay for the equipment and clothes that they need once they give birth. If you are worried, just sit down and make a list of everything you need. You can also see if there are some items that you can borrow from your family or friends.

You do not have to buy everything on your list. You will need baskets and cribs only for a short duration, and you can borrow these items from your friends. You can also buy many of the items second-hand. If you do not want to buy these products online, you can ask a friend to help you out.

If you are constantly worried about money and about how you are going to give your baby a good start, you should speak to your doctor or midwife. You can also get in touch with the local children's center to see where you can get some of the items that you are looking for. You can check with your employer if you are eligible for any programs at work and see if there are any benefits that you can claim. It is important that you ensure that you get your full maternity leave and pay. Speak to your human resources manager and understand the different benefits and support that your employer is offering.

Attend Complementary Therapies

One of the best ways to de-stress is to take a massage. You can ask your partner to give you a lower back massage, and if they do not know how to do it show them a video to help them understand the same. You can also ask them to give you a relaxation massage. If you do not want their help, you can learn how you can give yourself a foot massage. Many beauty salons and spas provide different pregnancy massage treatments. You must ensure that the person giving you the massage is qualified to work with pregnant women. Some studies show that aromatherapy helps to reduce anxiety. It also helps you feel relaxed and calm.

Be Mindful

Mindfulness is one of the best ways to connect with your surroundings. You can enjoy every moment, and not think about negative things. This means that you will need to spend all your energy and focus only on those moments in life where you are ecstatic, like when you first felt your baby kick. Research shows that practicing mindfulness helps to ease worry, depression, stress and anxiety in pregnant women. Let us look at some tips you can use to be mindful every day in your life:

- Always pay attention to the scents, sounds, sights and any other sensation around you when you are going about your day. It will be hard to do this at all times, so take some time out every day and focus on everything that you are experiencing.

- If you have the same routine every day, you can stop and look at the familiar things around you. You should always try to do something new every day, like take a different route, walk to a different shop or sit in a different place every time you step out for a walk.

- Always take some time out to focus on your thoughts and pay attention to the flow of your thoughts. Let your mind drift and see how your thoughts flow. Make sure that you give each thought or feeling a name and try to identify some pattern between those thoughts and feelings.

- You can also practice mindfulness meditation. You will need to close your eyes and focus only on your breathing or the sounds around you. If you find your mind wandering, you should bring it back.

Treat Yourself

One of the best ways to relax is to laugh. Try to read a good novel, watch some funny videos or movies, play funny games with your partner or meet up with your friends. You should spend on all the beauty treatments during your pregnancy.

What If You Are Still Stressed?

You should speak to your doctor or midwife if your stress levels are too high. The minute you start to feel overwhelmed, you should meet your doctor. You could be suffering either from depression or anxiety, or you may need some help to stop thinking negatively. We all need someone to help us sort our thoughts out.

Your doctor or midwife may ask you to attend some support group meetings or may refer you to a psychotherapist or counselor. You may also be asked to undergo cognitive behavior therapy depending on the severity of your stress. Your doctor or midwife may give you some strategies that you can use to help you tackle the anxiety or depression.

If you are taking any medication for any mental health condition like depression, you must ensure that you do not stop taking it abruptly. Ask your doctor what the risks of taking this medication are during your pregnancy. You may need to continue to take the medication or may be asked to undergo cognitive behavior therapy.

You may feel that your stress is not too bad, and that you are not anxious or depression. If it still bothers you, you should speak to your doctor or midwife during any of your appointments. When you get the right help, you can cope with stress during pregnancy and even after you give birth.

Chapter Four: Your Body after Pregnancy

As mentioned earlier, your body goes through many changes when you give birth, and these changes can be both emotional and physical. It is important for you to learn more about any postpartum discomforts that you may have after birth and see what you can do to overcome that discomfort. Before you treat any discomfort that you may be feeling, you should speak to your doctor or midwife. There are some medicines that you should not take when you are breastfeeding. Make sure that you attend all your checkups even if you do not feel any different. There are some conditions that will need to be treated immediately after you give birth.

Changes in Your Body A Few Weeks after You Give Birth

Your body will go through many changes after you have a baby. You will notice that your body went through numerous changes during pregnancy, and your body worked very hard to keep you and your baby healthy and safe. Your body will change again after you give birth. Some of the changes that your body goes through are physical, like your breasts growing larger and being full of milk, while others are emotional, like stress.

It is normal to be slightly uncomfortable after you give birth, and it is normal for your body to change. That said, some of the changes and discomfort that you feel could be symptoms of health issues, and you should treat these changes immediately. Ensure that you go for all your checkups even if you think you are okay. It is important to visit the doctor regularly after you give birth to ensure that you are recovering well. Your doctor can spot any irregularities and inform you immediately. It is important that you take care of yourself since new mothers are at a higher risk of developing some life-threatening complications a few weeks after they give birth.

What is perineum soreness?

The area between your rectum and vagina is called the perineum. This area will stretch, and may tear, during labor and birth. This area is often very sore after you give birth and could be sorer if you choose to have an episiotomy. An episiotomy is a cut made in the perineum to help the baby come out. If you do feel sore, you can try the following:

- Perform some Kegel exercises. Kegel exercises will strengthen the muscles in the pelvic area. When you do this exercise, you should squeeze the muscles in your pelvic region that you use to stop yourself from passing urine. You should hold these muscles tight for at least ten seconds and release them. Repeat this exercise ten times and perform the exercise at least thrice a day.
- Place a cold pack on the perineum. You can either buy a cold pack and place it in your freezer or wrap ice in a towel and use it as a cold pack.
- Always sit on a donut-shaped pillow or cushion.
- Always take a warm bath.
- You may develop infections while the episiotomy is healing. Make sure that you wipe your pelvic region after you go to the bathroom to prevent the development of any infection.
- Speak to your doctor to understand how you can deal with the soreness.

What are afterbirth pains?

Your uterus would have expanded during pregnancy to provide enough space to your baby, and it will need to shrink to its regular size once you give birth. When your uterus is shrinking, you will feel some cramps in your belly. These cramps will go away in a few days. When you are pregnant, your uterus will weigh close to 2.5 ounces, and is hard and round. When your uterus shrinks back to its size, it will only weigh two ounces. If the pain is unbearable, you can ask your doctor to prescribe some medication to ease the pain.

Changes in the Body after a Cesarean

If you choose to give birth through a C-section or cesarean, your doctor will make a cut in your uterus and belly to help the baby come out. This is a major surgery, and your body will take some time to recover. You may be extremely tired during the first few days after you give birth because you may have lost a lot of blood during the procedure. The cut on your belly will be sore.

Here are some tips to help you deal with the pain and the changes:

- If you feel a lot of pain, you can ask the doctor to provide you with some pain medication. Never take a medicine without checking with your doctor.
- Since you will be tired, you should ask your partners, friends or family to help you with the baby.
- Try to get enough rest. Make sure that you sleep when your baby sleeps. This means that you should sleep during the day too.
- Never lift any object that is heavier than your baby.
- Do not squat.
- Always support your belly when you are feeding your baby.
- Replace the fluids in your body by drinking enough water.

Vaginal Discharge

Your body will need to get rid of all the tissue and blood that was present inside your uterus to protect your baby. It will need to remove these from the body, and this discharge is called lochia or vaginal discharge. You will see that the discharge is bright red and can have some blood clots in it. This will only happen for a few days after you give birth. Over time, the flow will reduce, and the discharge will become lighter. You may have this discharge for a few weeks or a month. You will need to wear sanitary pads until the flow stops.

Breast Engorgement

A few weeks after you give birth, your breasts will begin to fill with milk. They will feel very sore and tender, but this discomfort will go away quickly when you start feeding your baby regularly. If you do not want to breastfeed, the tenderness will last until your breasts will stop making milk. This will happen in a few days. You can use the tips below to help you during this phase:

- Always feed your baby. Never take a long break between feedings and do not miss a feeding. You must never skip feeding your baby in the night.
- You should always remove some milk from your breasts before you feed your baby. You can do this by pressing your

breasts with your hand or through a breast pump.

- Always lay on warm towels or take a warm shower to help the milk flow. If your breasts are very tender, you should use cold packs.
- When you are not feeding, your breasts may lead. To prevent your clothes from getting wet, you should wear nursing pads in your bra.
- If your breasts are painful and are still swollen, you should speak to your doctor to understand why.
- If you do not want to breastfeed, you should wear a supportive and firm bra.

Nipple Pain

You may feel some pain around your nipples when you breastfeed. You will feel this pain during the first few days, and the pain worsens if your nipples begin to crack. Let us look at some tips to help you handle the pain:

- Speak to a lactation consultant or your doctor and ensure that your baby is sucking on your nipples in the right way.

-   Ask your doctor to prescribe some cream that you can use on your nipples.
-   After you are done feeding, massage your nipples and breasts with some milk, and do not cover your breasts until they are dry.

Swelling

Many women will have some swelling in their face, hand and feet during pregnancy, and this is caused due to the accumulation of the excess fluid in your body. It will take time for this swelling to reduce even after you give birth. Use the following tips to help you with easing the swelling:

-   Always lie on your left side when you are sleeping or resting.
-   Pull your feet up and sit.
-   Make sure that you wear loose clothes and always stay cool.
-   Drink a lot of water.

Hemorrhoids

The veins around the anus can begin to pain or may be swollen. These veins are called hemorrhoids, and they may bleed or hurt after you give birth. It is common to have hemorrhoids during pregnancy and after you give birth. Let us look at some tips that will help you deal with hemorrhoids:

- Always take a warm water bath.
- Speak to your doctor and see if you can use a cream or spray to ease the pain.
- Consume foods like whole-grain cereals or bread, vegetables and fruit to increase your fiber intake.
- Drink a lot of water.
- Never strain yourself too much when you are pooping.

Constipation

There are times when you find it difficult to pass stools because you do not have any bowel movements. This is called constipation. You will find that you are constipated for a few days after giving birth. If you have constipation, use the following tips:

- Always consume foods that are rich in fiber.
- Drink a lot of fluids.
- Speak to your provider to understand what medicine you can take to ease the constipation.

Urinary Problems after Giving Birth

You may have a burning sensation or feel pain when you urinate after you give birth. There may be times when you want to urinate, but you are unable to while there will be times when you want to stop urinating, but you cannot. This condition is called incontinence and it will go away when your muscles in the pelvic region become strong again. If you are having trouble with urinating, use the tips given below:

- Drink plenty of water.
- Always leave a tap running when you want to go to the bathroom.
- Take a warm bath.
- Speak to your provider if the pain continues.

Sweating After Giving Birth

You may sweat too much at night after you give birth, and this is caused because the hormones in your body are changing. Wear loose clothes when you go to bed and try to avoid covering yourself with too many blankets when you go to sleep. You should also sleep on a towel if you want to keep the sheets and pillow dry.

How to Lose Weight after Giving Birth?

You will lose at least ten pounds of weight immediately after you give birth and will lose a few more pounds in the first week. It is a good idea to reach your ideal weight during this time regardless of how much weight you may have gained during your pregnancy. You should be active and consume a healthy diet, which will help to boost your energy levels. You will feel much better if you have enough energy. You will not develop any health conditions, like high blood pressure and diabetes, if you reach a healthy weight. If you want to have another baby in the future, it is important that you reach your ideal weight before your second pregnancy. Let us look at some tips you can use to reach a healthy weight:

- Speak to your doctor about the weight you have gained and ask them to help you identify a way to reach your ideal weight.
- Limit your intake of processed foods and sweets.
- Follow a healthy diet.
- Drink a lot of water.
- Ask your doctor to help you understand how active you can be after you have given birth, especially if you have had a cesarean. Always begin slowly and increase the activity over time. You can swim or walk, but make sure that you stay active.
- You do burn a few calories when you breastfeed.
- Never try to lose too much weight because your body will need nutrients to heal. You will also reduce the supply of milk in your breasts if you lose weight too fast.
- You may not lose weight quickly, and this is fine. Do not be upset about it. Your body will take time to get back in shape. It is important that you stay fit for a longer time than worry about getting into shape immediately after you give birth.

What skin changes can happen after giving birth?

You will have some stretch marks on your abdomen and belly since you skin stretched when you were pregnant. Some women also have stretch marks on their bottom, thighs and hips. These stretch marks will not disappear after you give birth, but they will fade. You can apply different lotions or creams on your skin. That being said, these lotions and creams do not make these marks go away. They merely help to reduce the itching around those marks.

What hair changes can happen after giving birth?

You may have noticed that your hair was fuller and thicker during your pregnancy, and this is because the hormone levels in your body reduced hair loss. After you give birth, you will notice that your hair has started to thin out, and you may lose a lot of hair. You will stop losing hair after six months, and your hair will return to its normal volume in a year. If you want to avoid losing hair, you can do the following:

- Consume large quantities of fruit and vegetables. The nutrients will protect your hair and help it grow.
- Always be gentle with your hair. Do not wear braids, rollers or tight ponytails. These will stress your hair and pull it out.
- Always set your hair dryer to cool when you use it.

When do you get your period again after pregnancy?

Your period will start between the sixth and eighth week after you have given birth. This only happens when you are not breastfeeding. If you are feeding, your period will not start for a few months. Some women do not get their period until they stop feeding. If your period returns, it will not be the same as it was before your pregnancy. It could either be shorter or longer. It will soon return to how it used to be before your pregnancy.

When can you get pregnant again?

Doctors and physicians recommend that women give their body at least six weeks to heal after they give birth. This means that they can only have sex after six weeks. Even when your body is ready to have sex, you must be careful since you can get pregnant very easily. You will need to ovulate before you get your next period, and it will take your body at least six weeks before it can ovulate.

If you do not want to get pregnant again, you should use birth control, like intrauterine devices, pills, condoms and implants. Speak to your doctor or midwife about the birth control that you should use, especially if you are feeding. Some birth controls will reduce the supply of milk.

It is always a good idea to wait for at least eighteen months before you become pregnant again. When you increase the time between your pregnancies, you can reduce the risk of premature birth or low birth weight.

What Should You Do When You Feel Stressed Or Overwhelmed?

It is important for you to understand that your baby did not come with instructions. You will be overwhelmed and under a lot of stress when you are taking care of your baby. There is a lot that you will need to think about when it comes to a baby.

- Speak to your partner and let them know how you feel. Allow them to help you take care of the baby
- Ask your family and friends for help, and make sure that you let them know what it is exactly that you need them to do.
- Look for a support group with new mothers
- Always consume the right food, and make sure that you are always active
- Avoid consuming hard drugs, street drugs or alcohol. These substances will make it harder for you to handle the stress.

What are baby blues and postpartum depression?

Women sometimes are upset or sad after they have given birth to a baby. This phenomenon is called postpartum blues or baby blues. You may feel this way a few days after you give birth, and this feeling can last up to three weeks. You do not have to treat this feeling since it goes away on its own.

Postpartum depression, on the other hand, is a state of depression that women go into once they have given birth to their baby. If you suffer from postpartum depression, you will have strong feelings of worry, anxiety, tiredness and sadness, and these feelings will last for a very long time after you give birth. You will find it difficult to take care of yourself and your baby if you suffer from this type of depression. You will need to get yourself checked and treated. This is one of the most common forms of depression that women face after they give birth.

How to Deal With Baby Blues

- Try to sleep as much as you can
- Avoid any harmful drugs, street drugs and alcohol since these will affect your mood. There is a possibility that you may feel

worse after you consume these substances.
- Ask your partner to help you. You can also reach out to family and friends. Let them know what you feel and tell them how they can help you.
- Spend some time outside the house.
- Meet with other mothers.
- If you are upset or have these feelings for more than two weeks, speak to your doctor or midwife.

How to Deal With Postpartum Depression

- Speak to your doctor or midwife
- Understand what PPD is and what the risk factors are
- Learn more about the signs and symptoms
- Ask your doctor or midwife to help you understand how you can treat PPD

How can you handle going back to work or school?

It will definitely be hard for you to leave your baby at home all day with a family member, friend or a caregiver. It is also hard to trust the caregiver fully, and you and your partner may disagree on what is the best way to care for your child. You will be upset about the fact that you cannot stay at home with your baby. Let us see what you can do about this:

- Discuss how you want to care for your child with your partner. You should work on the finances and see how much you can spend. You should also talk to each other about the type of care you want to give your child. For instance, you can hire a caregiver who will come to your house and take care of the baby. Alternatively, you can drop your baby at a childcare center when you are away at work.
- You can ask family and friends to advise you on childcare. You can either use the same service as them or ask them if you can use the same person.
- If you want to use a childcare center, make sure that you obtain all the information about the people working at the center. You should also call other parents who use the center to see what they think about the center.
- You should ask your boss if it is okay for you to slowly ease into work. You can

work for a few hours from home at first, and then begin to work full time.

How can you and your partner get used to being new parents?

You and your partner are both getting used to having a third person in your house. Your partner is probably as nervous and stressed as you are, so make sure that you do not get irritated with them. Try to rely on each other and figure things out together. Let us look at what you both should do:

- Learn how to take care of your baby together. Take some baby-care classes or read some books to understand better.
- Do not try to do everything on your own. You should always talk to your partner and ask them to help with the baby.
- Learn to communicate. You should always talk about your feelings. This is the only way you can ensure that neither of you is frustrated.
- Always make time for each other. You can either go out for dinner or take a walk. Let someone take care of your baby for an hour.

- You should be open with your partner
  about sex, and make sure that you both
  are aware of when you can have sex again.
  If you do not want to speak directly to
  your partner about this, ask your doctor
  or midwife to speak to them.

Conclusion

Thank you for purchasing the book.

Pregnancy is a time of joy, but it is also a time when you will experience numerous changes in your body and in your life. It is important to learn how to deal with these changes. Over the course of the book, you will gather information about what causes stress during pregnancy and what you can do to overcome that stress, among other information.

I hope you have a calm and peaceful pregnancy and wish you luck on your journey.

Sources

https://www.womansday.com/health-fitness/womens-health/g2934/toxic-chemicals-to-avoid-when-pregnant/

https://www.babycentre.co.uk/a552044/11-ways-to-survive-stress-in-pregnancy

https://www.babycentre.co.uk/a547370/the-basics-of-good-sleep-in-pregnancy

https://www.self.com/story/8-important-things-women-forget-to-do-after-having-a-baby

https://www.marchofdimes.org/pregnancy/your-body-after-baby-the-first-6-weeks.aspx

www.ingramcontent.com/pod-product-compliance
Lightning Source LLC
Chambersburg PA
CBHW061732250726
48657CB00002B/884